THE CROHN'S DISEASE DIET BIBLE

How To Manage Crohn's Disease With A Beginner's Diet: Finding The Right Balance Between Comfort And Nutrition For Digestive Health

CRUE GAGE

Copyright © 2024 By Crue Gage

All Rights Reserved.

Table of Contents

Introductory 5

CHAPTER ONE 9

  Symptoms And Diagnosis 9

  Macronutrients: Carbohydrates, Proteins, And Fats 12

  Micronutrients: Vitamins And Minerals 16

CHAPTER TWO 20

  The Role Of Fiber In Digestive Health ... 20

  Foods To Include 23

  Foods To Avoid 27

CHAPTER THREE 31

  Meal Planning And Preparation 31

  Maintaining Nutritional Balance 39

  Breakfast Recipes 43

  Lunch Recipes 48

  Dinner Recipes 53

  Snacks And Smoothies Recipes 59

CHAPTER FOUR 64

Coping Strategies & Lifestyle Adjustments 64

Conclusion 68

THE END 70

Introductory

Crohn's disease is a form of inflammatory bowel disease (IBD) that results in chronic inflammation of the gastrointestinal tract. It can affect any part of the digestive system, from the pharynx to the anus; however, it is most frequently observed in the ileum (the final section of the small intestine) and the colon. Abdominal pain, diarrhea, fatigue, malnutrition, and weight loss are potential symptoms.

The precise cause is unknown; however, it is believed to be a result of a combination of genetic, environmental, and immune factors. Medications, lifestyle modifications, and occasionally surgery are employed to alleviate symptoms and reduce inflammation in the course of treatment.

Diet plays a crucial role in managing Crohn's disease, though individual needs can vary significantly. Here are some key points regarding the importance of diet for those with Crohn's:

• **Symptom Management**: Certain foods may trigger symptoms like diarrhea, cramping, or bloating. Keeping a food diary can help identify personal triggers.

• **Nutritional Balance**: Crohn's can affect nutrient absorption, leading to deficiencies. A well-balanced diet rich in vitamins and minerals is essential to combat potential deficiencies.

• **Fiber Intake**: While fiber is important for gut health, during flare-ups, a low-fiber diet may be recommended to reduce irritation. Once in remission, a gradual reintroduction of fiber can be beneficial.

- **Hydration**: Diarrhea can lead to dehydration, making adequate fluid intake vital.

- **Small, Frequent Meals**: Eating smaller meals throughout the day can be easier on the digestive system than larger meals.

- **Specialized Diets**: Some people find relief with specific diets, such as low FODMAP, gluten-free, or specific carbohydrate diets, though it's important to consult a healthcare provider or dietitian before making significant changes.

- **Probiotics and Prebiotics**: These may help support gut health, but their effectiveness can vary by individual.

It's always best for individuals with Crohn's to work with healthcare professionals to create a personalized dietary plan that meets their unique needs.

CHAPTER ONE
Symptoms And Diagnosis

Symptoms of Crohn's Disease:

- **Abdominal Pain and Cramping**: Often located in the lower right abdomen.
- **Diarrhea**: Chronic and sometimes severe; can be bloody.
- **Weight Loss**: Due to reduced appetite or malabsorption of nutrients.
- **Fatigue**: Commonly linked to inflammation and nutrient deficiencies.
- **Fever**: May occur during flare-ups.
- **Mouth Sores**: Ulcers may develop in the mouth.
- **Nutritional Deficiencies**: Due to malabsorption.

- **Bloating and Gas**: Common digestive symptoms.

Diagnosis of Crohn's Disease:

- **Medical History and Physical Exam**: Discussion of symptoms and family history.
- **Blood Tests**: To check for anemia, inflammation markers (like C-reactive protein), and nutritional deficiencies.
- **Stool Tests**: To rule out infections and check for inflammation.

Imaging Studies:

- **CT or MRI Scans**: To visualize the intestines and detect inflammation or complications.

- **X-rays**: Sometimes used, especially after ingesting a contrast medium.

Endoscopy:

- **Colonoscopy**: To examine the entire colon and sometimes the ileum, allowing for biopsy collection.
- **Upper Endoscopy**: To check for involvement in the upper digestive tract.

A combination of these methods is often used to confirm a diagnosis and assess the extent of the disease. If you suspect you have Crohn's disease, it's important to consult a healthcare provider for proper evaluation and diagnosis.

Macronutrients: Carbohydrates, Proteins, And Fats

Macronutrients are the nutrients that provide energy and are essential for growth and maintenance of the body. They are divided into three main categories: carbohydrates, proteins, and fats. Here's a brief overview of each:

1. Carbohydrates:

• **Function**: Primary source of energy for the body. They are broken down into glucose, which fuels cells, especially in the brain and muscles.

Types:

• **Simple Carbohydrates**: Sugars that are quickly absorbed (e.g., glucose, fructose).

- **Complex Carbohydrates**: Starches and fibers that take longer to digest (e.g., whole grains, legumes, vegetables).

- **Sources**: Fruits, vegetables, grains, legumes, and dairy products.

- **Consideration for Crohn's**: Some individuals may need to limit high-fiber or high-sugar foods during flare-ups.

2. Proteins:

- **Function**: Essential for building and repairing tissues, producing enzymes and hormones, and supporting immune function.

- **Structure**: Made up of amino acids; there are 20 different amino acids, nine of which are essential (must be obtained through diet).

- **Sources**: Meat, poultry, fish, eggs, dairy products, legumes, nuts, and seeds.

- **Consideration for Crohn's**: Easily digestible proteins may be preferable during flare-ups; lean meats and plant-based sources can be beneficial.

3. Fats

- **Function**: Concentrated source of energy, important for cell structure, hormone production, and the absorption of fat-soluble vitamins (A, D, E, K).

Types:

- **Saturated Fats**: Usually solid at room temperature (e.g., butter, red meat). Should be consumed in moderation.

- **Unsaturated Fats**: Liquid at room temperature and considered healthier (e.g., olive oil, avocados, nuts).

- **Trans Fats**: Artificial fats found in some processed foods, should be avoided.

- **Sources**: Oils, nuts, seeds, fatty fish, and avocados.

- **Consideration for Crohn's**: Healthy fats are important, but individuals may need to monitor their intake based on personal tolerance.

When managing Crohn's disease, it's important to focus on a balanced intake of macronutrients that suit individual tolerance levels, especially during flare-ups. Consulting with a healthcare provider or dietitian can help create a tailored nutrition plan.

Micronutrients: Vitamins And Minerals

Micronutrients, which include vitamins and minerals, are essential for various bodily functions, including metabolism, immune function, and bone health. Unlike macronutrients, they are required in smaller amounts but are crucial for overall health. Here's an overview:

Vitamins

Vitamins are organic compounds that support numerous bodily processes. They are divided into two categories:

Water-Soluble Vitamins:

- **Vitamin C**: Important for immune function and collagen production.
- **B Vitamins** (e.g., B1, B2, B3, B6, B12, folate): Essential for energy metabolism, red blood cell

formation, and neurological function.

Fat-Soluble Vitamins:

• **Vitamins A, D, E, and K**: Important for vision, bone health, antioxidant functions, and blood clotting.

Minerals

Minerals are inorganic nutrients that play key roles in bodily functions. Some important ones include:

- **Calcium**: Vital for bone health and muscle function.
- **Iron**: Essential for red blood cell production and oxygen transport.
- **Magnesium**: Important for muscle and nerve function, as well as energy production.

- **Zinc**: Supports immune function and wound healing.

Micronutrients and Crohn's Disease

Individuals with Crohn's disease may be at risk for micronutrient deficiencies due to:

- Malabsorption in the intestines.
- Reduced dietary intake during flare-ups.
- Increased nutritional needs during periods of inflammation.

Common Deficiencies:

- **Iron**: Often due to blood loss or malabsorption.
- **Vitamin B12**: May be poorly absorbed, especially if the ileum is affected.

- **Calcium and Vitamin D**: Important for bone health, especially if corticosteroids are used.

It's essential for individuals with Crohn's disease to monitor their micronutrient intake, potentially through dietary adjustments or supplementation, under the guidance of a healthcare provider or dietitian. Regular blood tests can help identify deficiencies.

CHAPTER TWO
The Role Of Fiber In Digestive Health

Fiber plays a vital role in digestive health and overall well-being. Here's how it contributes:

Types of Fiber:

• **Soluble Fiber**: Dissolves in water, forming a gel-like substance. It can help lower cholesterol levels and stabilize blood sugar.

• **Sources**: Oats, legumes, fruits (like apples and citrus), and some vegetables.

• **Insoluble Fiber**: Does not dissolve in water and adds bulk to stool, helping food move through the digestive tract.

• **Sources**: Whole grains, nuts, seeds, and the skins of fruits and vegetables.

Benefits of Fiber for Digestive Health:

• **Promotes Regular Bowel Movements**: Insoluble fiber helps prevent constipation by adding bulk to the stool and speeding up transit time through the intestines.

• **Supports Gut Health**: Fiber can act as a prebiotic, providing food for beneficial gut bacteria, which helps maintain a healthy microbiome.

• **May Help Prevent Digestive Disorders**: A high-fiber diet is linked to a reduced risk of developing conditions like diverticulitis and colorectal cancer.

• **Aids in Weight Management**: Fiber-rich foods are often more filling, which can help control appetite and reduce overall calorie intake.

Considerations for Crohn's Disease

- **During Flare-Ups**: Some individuals with Crohn's may need to limit high-fiber foods, especially insoluble fiber, to reduce irritation in the intestines.

- **In Remission**: Once in remission, gradually reintroducing fiber can be beneficial for digestive health.

General Recommendations

- Aim for a balanced intake of both soluble and insoluble fiber.
- Increase fiber intake gradually to allow the digestive system to adjust.
- Stay hydrated, as fiber works best when paired with adequate fluid intake.

Always consult with a healthcare provider or dietitian to tailor fiber intake based on individual needs and health conditions.

Foods To Include

When managing digestive health, especially for conditions like Crohn's disease, it's essential to choose foods that are gentle on the digestive system and provide essential nutrients. Here's a list of foods to consider including:

Foods to Include

Low-Fiber Fruits:

- Bananas
- Apples (without skin)
- Canned peaches or pears
- Melons

Cooked Vegetables:

- Carrots
- Zucchini
- Spinach
- Squash
- Potatoes (without skin)

Whole Grains (in moderation, depending on tolerance):

- Oats (preferably cooked)
- White rice
- Quinoa (if tolerated)

Lean Proteins:

- Chicken and turkey (skinless)
- Fish and seafood
- Eggs
- Tofu
- Smooth nut butters (if tolerated)

Dairy Alternatives (if lactose intolerant):

- Lactose-free milk or yogurt
- Almond milk or soy milk

Healthy Fats:

- Olive oil
- Avocado (in moderation)
- Nut oils (in moderation)

Low-FODMAP Foods (if sensitive to fermentable carbs):

- Certain fruits (like blueberries)
- Certain vegetables (like bell peppers and carrots)

Tips:

• **Cooking Methods**: Cooking foods can help make them easier to digest (steaming, boiling, or baking).

- **Portion Sizes**: Smaller, more frequent meals can be easier on the digestive system.

- **Stay Hydrated**: Drink plenty of fluids, especially if increasing fiber intake.

Always consult with a healthcare provider or dietitian to create a personalized eating plan tailored to your specific needs and symptoms.

Foods To Avoid

When managing digestive health, especially with conditions like Crohn's disease, certain foods may exacerbate symptoms. Here's a list of foods to consider avoiding:

Foods to Avoid

High-Fiber Foods (during flare-ups):

- Whole grains (e.g., whole wheat bread, brown rice)
- Raw fruits and vegetables, especially with skins or seeds
- Legumes (beans, lentils, chickpeas)
- Nuts and seeds

Fatty and Fried Foods:

- Fried foods (e.g., fried chicken, French fries)

- High-fat dairy products (e.g., whole milk, cream, cheese)

Spicy Foods:

- Hot peppers, spicy sauces, and heavily seasoned dishes can irritate the digestive tract.

Caffeine and Alcohol:

- Caffeinated beverages (e.g., coffee, energy drinks) and alcoholic drinks can stimulate the gut and lead to discomfort.

Processed and Sugary Foods:

- Sugary snacks (e.g., candies, pastries) and processed foods high in preservatives and additives can lead to gastrointestinal distress.

Certain Dairy Products (if lactose intolerant):

- Milk, soft cheeses, and ice cream may cause bloating or diarrhea.

Artificial Sweeteners:

- Some people may find that sugar alcohols (e.g., sorbitol, mannitol) can cause bloating and gas.

Tips:

- **Keep a Food Diary**: Tracking what you eat and your symptoms can help identify personal triggers.
- **Reintroduce Foods Gradually**: If you want to test the tolerance of certain foods, do so one at a time and monitor your body's response.

Always consult with a healthcare provider or dietitian to tailor dietary choices based on individual symptoms and health status.

CHAPTER THREE
Meal Planning And Preparation

Meal planning and preparation can be especially beneficial for managing digestive health and conditions like Crohn's disease. Here are some tips to help you get started:

<u>Meal Planning Tips:</u>

- **Assess Personal Tolerances**: Keep a food diary to identify which foods trigger symptoms and which are well-tolerated.
- **Balanced Meals**: Aim for a balance of macronutrients (carbohydrates, proteins, and fats) and include micronutrient-rich foods.
- **Plan for Flare-Ups**: Have easy-to-digest foods on hand (e.g., cooked

vegetables, lean proteins) for times when symptoms worsen.

- **Portion Control**: Opt for smaller, more frequent meals to reduce digestive strain.
- **Weekly Meal Prep**: Set aside time each week to prepare meals in advance, making it easier to stick to your dietary plan.

Meal Preparation Tips:

- **Batch Cooking**: Prepare large quantities of soups, stews, or casseroles that can be portioned and frozen for later use.
- **Simple Cooking Methods**: Use gentle cooking methods like steaming, boiling, or baking to make foods easier to digest.

- **Prepare Snacks**: Have healthy snacks ready (e.g., yogurt, bananas, or nut butter) to avoid unhealthy choices.
- **Read Labels**: If using packaged foods, check labels for additives, sugars, and fiber content.
- **Hydration**: Always keep water or clear fluids available to stay hydrated, especially if increasing fiber intake.

Sample Meal Plan

Breakfast:

- Scrambled eggs with spinach (cooked)
- Oatmeal (cooked) with banana

Lunch:

- Grilled chicken breast with steamed carrots and zucchini
- Quinoa (if tolerated) or white rice

Snack:

- Lactose-free yogurt or a banana

Dinner:

- Baked fish (e.g., salmon) with mashed potatoes (without skin) and cooked green beans

Evening Snack:

- Smooth nut butter on a rice cake or a small serving of applesauce
- Always adjust the meal plan based on personal preferences and tolerances, and consult with a healthcare provider or dietitian for individualized advice.

Managing Flare-Ups

- Managing flare-ups of Crohn's disease requires a proactive approach to minimize symptoms and support recovery. Here are some strategies:

Dietary Strategies:

- **Stick to Easily Digestible Foods**: Focus on low-fiber, bland foods during flare-ups, such as cooked vegetables, lean proteins, and refined grains.
- **Stay Hydrated**: Drink plenty of fluids, especially water or clear broths, to prevent dehydration, particularly if experiencing diarrhea.
- **Small, Frequent Meals**: Eating smaller meals throughout the day

can reduce digestive strain and help manage symptoms.
- **Avoid Trigger Foods**: Identify and steer clear of foods that typically exacerbate symptoms, such as spicy foods, high-fiber foods, and fatty or fried items.

Lifestyle Strategies:

- **Rest**: Ensure adequate rest to help the body recover during a flare-up. Fatigue can worsen symptoms.
- **Stress Management**: Practice stress-reducing techniques like deep breathing, meditation, or gentle yoga, as stress can trigger flare-ups.
- **Monitor Symptoms**: Keep a symptom diary to track flare-up triggers, duration, and severity.

This can help in discussing patterns with a healthcare provider.

Medical Management

- **Follow Prescribed Treatment:** Adhere to medications as prescribed by your healthcare provider, including anti-inflammatory drugs, immunosuppressants, or corticosteroids.
- **Consult Your Healthcare Provider:** If symptoms worsen or don't improve, reach out for guidance on adjusting treatment plans or exploring additional options.
- **Consider Supplements:** If experiencing nutritional

deficiencies, discuss the possibility of supplements (like vitamins or minerals) with a healthcare professional.

When to Seek Help:

- Seek medical attention if you experience:
- Severe abdominal pain
- Persistent diarrhea (especially if bloody)
- High fever
- Signs of dehydration (e.g., excessive thirst, dry mouth, reduced urination)
- Unexplained weight loss

Managing flare-ups effectively involves a combination of dietary adjustments, lifestyle changes, and medical care. Always consult with a healthcare provider for personalized advice and treatment options.

Maintaining Nutritional Balance

Maintaining nutritional balance is crucial for overall health, especially for individuals with conditions like Crohn's disease. Here are some key strategies to achieve this:

1. Diverse Food Choices:

- **Variety**: Incorporate a wide range of foods from all food groups (fruits, vegetables, grains, proteins, and healthy fats) to ensure a comprehensive intake of nutrients.

- **Colorful Plate**: Aim for a colorful plate, as different colors often represent different nutrients.

2. Monitor Macronutrients:

- **Carbohydrates**: Choose complex carbohydrates (like cooked grains and starchy vegetables) for sustained energy, especially if fiber tolerance allows.

- **Proteins**: Include lean protein sources (chicken, fish, tofu, eggs) to support tissue repair and muscle health.

- **Fats**: Opt for healthy fats (olive oil, avocados, nuts) while limiting saturated and trans fats.

3. Micronutrient Awareness:

- Be mindful of essential vitamins and minerals that may be deficient, especially iron, calcium, vitamin D, and vitamin B12.

- Consider fortified foods or supplements as needed, in consultation with a healthcare provider.

4. Meal Planning:

- **Balanced Meals**: Aim for balanced meals that include a source of protein, healthy fats, and carbohydrates.

- **Snack Smart**: Choose nutritious snacks (like yogurt, fruit, or nuts) to help meet energy and nutrient needs.

5. Hydration:

- Drink plenty of fluids, especially water, to support digestion and overall health. Consider electrolyte-replenishing beverages if experiencing diarrhea.

6. Limit Processed Foods:

- Minimize intake of processed and sugary foods, as they can lack essential nutrients and contribute to digestive discomfort.

7. Listen to Your Body:

- Pay attention to how different foods affect your symptoms and overall well-being. Adjust your diet accordingly.

8. Consult Professionals:

- Work with a registered dietitian or healthcare provider who specializes in digestive health to tailor a nutritional plan that meets your specific needs.

By focusing on these strategies, you can help maintain nutritional balance and support your overall health while managing Crohn's disease or other digestive issues.

Breakfast Recipes

Here are some easy and nutritious breakfast recipes that are gentle on the digestive system, especially suitable for individuals managing Crohn's disease:

1. Scrambled Eggs with Spinach

Ingredients:

- 2 eggs
- A handful of fresh spinach (cooked)
- Salt and pepper to taste
- Olive oil or butter

Instructions:

- Heat olive oil or butter in a non-stick pan over medium heat.

- Add spinach and sauté until wilted.
- Whisk eggs in a bowl and pour them into the pan.
- Stir gently until eggs are cooked to your liking. Season with salt and pepper.

2. Oatmeal with Banana

Ingredients:

- 1/2 cup rolled oats
- 1 cup water or milk (or a milk alternative)
- 1 small banana, sliced
- A drizzle of honey or maple syrup (optional)

Instructions:

- In a pot, combine oats and water/milk. Bring to a boil.

- Reduce heat and simmer for about 5 minutes, stirring occasionally.
- Once thickened, remove from heat and top with banana slices and a drizzle of honey or syrup if desired.

3. Smoothie Bowl:

Ingredients:

- 1 banana
- 1/2 cup yogurt (lactose-free if needed)
- A handful of spinach (optional)
- A small amount of almond milk (or water) for blending
- Toppings: sliced fruits, a sprinkle of cinnamon, or nut butter

Instructions:

- Blend banana, yogurt, spinach, and almond milk until smooth.
- Pour into a bowl and add your favorite toppings.

4. Rice Cakes with Nut Butter

Ingredients:

- 1-2 rice cakes
- Smooth nut butter (like almond or peanut butter)
- Sliced banana or applesauce

Instructions:

- Spread nut butter on rice cakes.
- Top with banana slices or a spoonful of applesauce for added flavor.

5. Yogurt Parfait:

Ingredients:

- 1 cup yogurt (lactose-free if needed)
- A small handful of soft berries (like blueberries or strawberries)
- A drizzle of honey (optional)

Instructions:

- Layer yogurt with berries in a bowl or cup.
- Drizzle with honey if desired for sweetness.

These recipes are nutritious, easy to prepare, and can be adjusted based on individual dietary needs and tolerances. Enjoy!

Lunch Recipes

Here are some simple and nutritious lunch recipes that are easy on the digestive system, especially suitable for individuals managing Crohn's disease:

1. Quinoa and Chicken Salad

Ingredients:

- 1 cup cooked quinoa
- 1 cooked chicken breast, shredded
- 1/2 cup cooked carrots (chopped)
- 1/4 cup cucumber (peeled and diced)
- Olive oil and lemon juice for dressing
- Salt and pepper to taste

Instructions:

- In a bowl, combine cooked quinoa, shredded chicken, carrots, and cucumber.
- Drizzle with olive oil and lemon juice, and season with salt and pepper. Mix well and serve.

2. Vegetable Soup

Ingredients:

- 2 cups low-sodium chicken or vegetable broth
- 1 cup chopped cooked vegetables (carrots, zucchini, spinach)
- 1/2 cup cooked lentils (optional)
- Salt and pepper to taste
- A pinch of dried herbs (like thyme or basil)

Instructions:

- In a pot, bring broth to a simmer.

- Add cooked vegetables and lentils (if using) and simmer for 10-15 minutes.
- Season with salt, pepper, and herbs. Serve warm.

3. Turkey and Avocado Wrap

Ingredients:

- Whole wheat or gluten-free wrap
- Sliced turkey breast
- 1/4 avocado, sliced
- Spinach leaves
- A drizzle of olive oil or a light dressing

Instructions:

- Lay the wrap flat and layer with turkey, avocado, and spinach.
- Drizzle with olive oil or dressing, then roll tightly and slice in half.

4. Soft Scrambled Eggs with Toast

Ingredients:

- 2 eggs
- Salt and pepper to taste
- 1 slice of soft bread (gluten-free if needed)
- Olive oil or butter

Instructions:

- Whisk eggs with a pinch of salt and pepper.
- Heat olive oil or butter in a non-stick pan over low heat.
- Add eggs and stir gently until just set.
- Serve with a slice of toast on the side.

5. Hummus and Soft Veggie Plate

Ingredients:

- Store-bought or homemade hummus
- Soft cooked vegetables (carrots, zucchini, or bell peppers)
- Rice cakes or pita bread (if tolerated)

Instructions:

- Serve hummus in a bowl.
- Arrange soft-cooked vegetables and rice cakes or pita on the side for dipping.

These lunch recipes are not only nutritious but also easy to prepare and can be adjusted based on individual preferences and tolerances. Enjoy your meals!

Dinner Recipes

Here are some easy and nutritious dinner recipes that are gentle on the digestive system, especially suitable for those managing Crohn's disease:

1. Baked Salmon with Sweet Potatoes

Ingredients:

- 1 salmon fillet
- 1 medium sweet potato, peeled and cubed
- Olive oil
- Salt and pepper
- Fresh herbs (like dill or parsley, optional)

Instructions:

- Preheat the oven to 400°F (200°C).

- Toss sweet potato cubes with olive oil, salt, and pepper. Spread on a baking sheet and roast for about 20-25 minutes.
- Season the salmon with olive oil, salt, pepper, and herbs. Place it on the baking sheet during the last 12-15 minutes of roasting.
- Serve together once cooked.

2. Chicken and Rice Casserole

Ingredients:

- 1 cup cooked white rice
- 1 cooked chicken breast, shredded
- 1 cup low-sodium chicken broth
- 1/2 cup cooked carrots (chopped)
- 1/2 cup peas (optional)
- Salt and pepper to taste

Instructions:

- Preheat the oven to 350°F (175°C).
- In a baking dish, combine cooked rice, shredded chicken, broth, carrots, and peas.
- Season with salt and pepper. Mix well.
- Cover with foil and bake for 25-30 minutes until heated through.

3. Stir-Fried Tofu and Vegetables

Ingredients:

- 1 block of firm tofu, cubed
- 1 cup mixed soft vegetables (like bell peppers, zucchini, and spinach)
- Olive oil or sesame oil
- Soy sauce (low sodium)

- Ginger (fresh or powdered, optional)

Instructions:

- Heat oil in a pan over medium heat. Add tofu and sauté until golden brown.
- Add mixed vegetables and cook until soft.
- Stir in soy sauce and ginger (if using) and cook for another minute. Serve warm.

4. Creamy Pasta with Spinach

Ingredients:

- 1 cup pasta (white or gluten-free)
- 1 cup fresh spinach
- 1/2 cup cream or a dairy alternative
- Olive oil

- Salt and pepper to taste
- Grated Parmesan cheese (optional)

Instructions:

- Cook pasta according to package instructions.
- In a pan, heat olive oil and add spinach, cooking until wilted.
- Stir in cream and cooked pasta, mixing well. Season with salt, pepper, and Parmesan if desired.

5. Vegetable Omelette

Ingredients:

- 2 eggs
- 1/4 cup cooked vegetables (like bell peppers, spinach, or zucchini)
- Olive oil or butter
- Salt and pepper to taste

Instructions:

- Whisk eggs with salt and pepper.
- Heat oil or butter in a non-stick pan over medium heat. Add cooked vegetables.
- Pour eggs over the vegetables, cooking until set. Fold in half and serve warm.

These dinner recipes are nutritious, easy to prepare, and can be adjusted based on individual dietary needs and preferences. Enjoy!

Snacks And Smoothies Recipes

Here are some easy and nutritious snack and smoothie recipes that are gentle on the digestive system, especially suitable for individuals managing Crohn's disease:

Snack Recipes

Greek Yogurt with Honey:

- **Ingredients**: 1 cup Greek yogurt, drizzle of honey, soft berries (like blueberries).
- **Instructions**: Top Greek yogurt with honey and berries for a quick, protein-rich snack.

Rice Cakes with Nut Butter:

- **Ingredients**: Rice cakes, smooth almond or peanut butter, banana slices (optional).

- **Instructions**: Spread nut butter on rice cakes and top with banana slices if desired.

Cottage Cheese with Peaches:

- **Ingredients**: 1 cup cottage cheese, canned or fresh peach slices (peeled).
- **Instructions**: Mix peach slices into cottage cheese for a creamy and sweet snack.

Soft Veggie Sticks and Hummus:

- **Ingredients**: Soft-cooked carrot or cucumber sticks, hummus.
- **Instructions**: Serve soft-cooked veggie sticks with hummus for dipping.

Oatmeal Energy Bites

- **Ingredients**: 1 cup oats, 1/4 cup nut butter, 1/4 cup honey, and optional add-ins (like mini chocolate chips).
- **Instructions**: Mix all ingredients, form into small balls, and refrigerate until firm.

Smoothie Recipes

Banana Spinach Smoothie:

- **Ingredients**: 1 banana, 1 cup spinach, 1/2 cup yogurt (lactose-free if needed), 1/2 cup almond milk.
- **Instructions**: Blend all ingredients until smooth. Adjust thickness by adding more almond milk if desired.

Berry Yogurt Smoothie:

- **Ingredients**: 1/2 cup soft berries (like blueberries or strawberries), 1 cup yogurt, 1/2 banana, 1/2 cup water or milk.
- **Instructions**: Blend until smooth and serve chilled.

Peach Oat Smoothie:

- **Ingredients**: 1 cup canned peaches (drained), 1/4 cup oats, 1/2 cup yogurt, 1/2 cup water or almond milk.
- **Instructions**: Blend all ingredients until smooth. Add ice for a chilled smoothie.

Mango Coconut Smoothie:

- **Ingredients**: 1 cup frozen mango chunks, 1/2 cup coconut milk, 1/2 banana.
- **Instructions**: Blend until creamy. Adjust thickness with more coconut milk as needed.

Avocado Green Smoothie

- **Ingredients**: 1/2 avocado, 1 banana, 1 cup spinach, 1/2 cup yogurt, 1/2 cup water or almond milk.
- **Instructions**: Blend until smooth and creamy.

These snack and smoothie recipes are easy to prepare and can be adjusted based on individual preferences and tolerances. Enjoy!

CHAPTER FOUR
Coping Strategies & Lifestyle Adjustments

Coping with Crohn's disease involves both mental and physical strategies to manage symptoms and maintain a good quality of life. Here are some effective coping strategies and lifestyle adjustments:

Coping Strategies:

• Learn about Crohn's disease, its symptoms, and treatments. Understanding your condition can empower you to make informed decisions about your health.

• Join support groups or online communities where you can share experiences and tips with others who have Crohn's disease.

- Talk to friends, family, and healthcare providers about your needs and challenges. Open communication can help foster understanding and support.

- Engage in mindfulness techniques such as meditation, deep breathing, or yoga to help reduce stress and improve mental well-being.

- Consider working with a therapist or counselor, especially if you're struggling with anxiety or depression related to your condition.

<u>Lifestyle Adjustments</u>

- Follow a nutritious diet tailored to your needs. Focus on easy-to-digest foods, monitor fiber intake, and stay hydrated.

- Incorporate gentle exercise like walking, swimming, or yoga into your routine.

Physical activity can improve mood and overall health.

• Prioritize getting enough sleep each night. Good sleep hygiene can help manage stress and improve overall health.

• Regular appointments with your healthcare provider can help monitor your condition and adjust treatment plans as needed.

• Identify stressors in your life and develop coping mechanisms to manage them, such as time management techniques or setting boundaries.

• Identify foods, situations, or activities that trigger your symptoms and try to limit or avoid them.

- Keep track of medications, appointments, and symptoms in a journal or app. This can help you stay on top of your health management.

- If traveling, plan ahead by packing necessary medications, snacks, and items that may help you manage symptoms on the go.

By incorporating these lifestyle modifications and coping strategies, you can more effectively manage Crohn's disease, resulting in a higher quality of life. Seek personalized guidance and assistance from your healthcare provider at all times.

Conclusion

A comprehensive strategy that includes lifestyle modifications, coping strategies, and dietary choices is necessary for the management of Crohn's disease.

Individuals can substantially improve their quality of life by emphasizing nutrition, maintaining connections with support networks, and implementing stress management strategies. In order to achieve effective management,

it is essential to educate oneself about the disease, monitor symptoms, and maintain open communication with healthcare providers. Furthermore, the adoption of moderate exercise, the prioritization of rest, and the identification of personal triggers can contribute to the overall well-being.

Remember, the experience of Crohn's disease is distinct for each individual. Consequently, it is crucial to customize these strategies to meet your individual requirements and seek the advice of healthcare professionals for personalized help. Navigating the obstacles of Crohn's disease and leading a fulfilling life is feasible with the appropriate resources and assistance.

THE END

www.ingramcontent.com/pod-product-compliance
Lightning Source LLC
Chambersburg PA
CBHW070214230526
45471CB00002B/947